COMPLETE GUIDE TO ANGIOPLASTY

Essential Manual To Understanding Procedures, Risks, Recovery, And Future Outlook In Cardiovascular Health, Updated Techniques, Stents, Recovery Tips, And More

DR. BRUNO HORAN

Copyright © 2023 by Dr. Bruno Horan

All rights reserved. Except for brief quotations embodied in critical reviews and certain other noncommercial uses permitted by copyright law, no part of this publication may be reproduced, distributed, or transmitted in any form or by any means, Including photocopying, recording, or other electronic or mechanical methods, without the prior written permission of the publisher.

Disclaimer:

The information provided in this book, is intended for general informational purposes only and should not be considered as professional advice.

The author has made every effort to ensure the accuracy of the information presented. However, readers are advised to consult with a qualified healthcare professional before attempting any herbal remedies or making significant changes to their wellness routine. Individual health conditions vary, and what may be suitable for one person may not be appropriate for another.

It is important to note that the author is not in any endorsement deal, partnership, or affiliation with any organization, brand, or company mentioned in this book. Any references to specific products or services are based on the author's personal experience or general knowledge and do not imply an endorsement or promotion of those products or services

Contents

CHAPTER ONE 17

  THE CARDIAC VASCULAR SYSTEM'S ANATOMY AND PHYSIOLOGY 17

    Heart's Structure 17

    The Role Of Blood Vessels 18

    Circulation Of Blood Through The Heart 19

    Arterial Blockages' Effects 20

CHAPTER TWO 21

  CAUSES OF ARTERIAL BLOCKAGES AND THEIR SYMPTOMS 21

    Risk Variables (Hereditary, Lifestyle) 22

    Signs Of Obstructed Arteries 23

    How Obstacles Arise 24

    What Separates Stable From Unstable Plaques ... 25

    The Value Of Early Identification 26

CHAPTER THREE 29

  DIAGNOSTIC METHODOLOGIES 29

    Non-Invasive Examinations (Stress Test, EKG) ... 29

    Imaging Methods (MRI, CT Angiography) 30

    Invasive Exams (Coronary Angiography) 31

Biomarkers And Blood Tests...................................32
  Interpreting The Findings Of A Diagnosis 33
CHAPTER FOUR 35
  EXPLAINED: THE ANGIOPLASTY PROCEDURE.......35
    Methodical Procedure 35
    Tools And Apparatus Employed 38
    What Takes Place Throughout The Process 40
CHAPTER FIVE 43
  DANGERS AND COMMITMENTS 43
    Typical Risks...43
    Uncommon Problems..44
    How Hazards Are Handled 45
    Breathing Problems Or Chest Pain 46
    When To Get Medical Assistance 47
CHAPTER SIX..49
  REPAY AND RESUMMATION 49
    Quick Post-Procedure Treatment 51
    Hospital Discharge Procedure...........................52
    Medication And Appointments For Follow-Up.......53
    Guidelines For Physical Activity.........................55

>   Mental And Emotional Assistance 56
> CHAPTER SEVEN 59
>   CHANGES IN LIFESTYLE AFTER ANGIOPLASTY 59
>   The Value Of A Balanced Diet 59
>   Follow Exercise Guidelines 61
>   Quitting Smoking 64
>   Stress Reduction 66
>   Routine Check-Ups With The Doctor 69
> CHAPTER EIGHT 73
>   QUESTIONS ASKED REGULARLY 73
>   What Is The Stent's Duration Of Use? 73
>   Can Blockages Happen Again? 74
>   How To Keep An Eye On Your Heart Health 76
>   Prognosis Over The Long Term And Quality Of Life
>   77

CONCERNING THIS BOOK

"Angioplasty" is a thorough manual that demystifies an important surgical operation that has transformed the way cardiovascular illnesses are treated. It starts with a precise explanation of angioplasty, outlining its historical development and outlining the several kinds that are currently accessible. Knowing who might benefit from angioplasty and its many advantages highlights the procedure's potential to save lives and paves the way for further research.

A good understanding of the cardiovascular system is necessary, and the heart's structure, blood vessels' functions, and the vital significance of coronary arteries are all covered in detail in this book. Understanding the effects of artery blockages and how blood travels through the heart is made easier by the text, which also explains why angioplasty is frequently required. The thorough explanations improve the reader's understanding of the subject matter by making difficult physiological and anatomical concepts understandable.

The main worry is arterial blockages, and the book explores the different risk factors that lead to this disorder, including genetic and lifestyle variables. It explains the biological mechanisms for plaque development as well as the symptoms that frequently accompany clogged arteries. Making the distinction between stable and unstable plaques highlights how important early diagnosis is for successful treatments and the avoidance of serious cardiac events.

A significant portion of the story is devoted to diagnostic techniques, which describe the variety of tests that are available to detect artery blockages. The book offers an extensive overview of sophisticated imaging techniques such as CT angiography and MRI, as well as non-invasive examinations including stress testing and EKGs. The reader's comprehension is further enhanced by the inclusion of invasive tests such as coronary angiography and the interpretation of diagnostic data, which emphasize the accuracy required in the diagnosis of cardiovascular problems.

The actual angioplasty method is described in great detail, including a step-by-step explanation of the steps, the instruments and equipment needed, and the vital role played by the interventional cardiologist. To make sure readers are prepared, the book gives a detailed description of the procedure's events as well as the crucial components of post-procedure care.

The book addresses the risks and complications of angioplasty, including typical and uncommon dangers such as bleeding, infection, stroke, and heart attack. It describes the warning indicators of problems that need to be seen by a doctor right away as well as how these risks are treated. To ensure that patients and their families are aware of potential obstacles and know when to seek assistance, this section is essential.

The book offers thorough instructions on post-operation care after an angioplasty, including the hospital discharge protocol, recovery and rehabilitation, required drugs, and follow-up appointments. Recognizing the entire nature of healing, it highlights the need for physical activity recommendations and provides insights into emotional and psychological assistance.

For long-term health following angioplasty, lifestyle modifications are critical, and the book emphasizes the need for stress management, quitting smoking, eating a balanced diet, and getting regular exercise. It also emphasizes how important it is for patients to get frequent check-ups to monitor their heart health and to help them adopt and maintain healthier lifestyles to avoid blockages in the future.

A section addressing frequently asked questions tackles common concerns that patients may have, including the impact on daily life, the likelihood of recurring blockages, and the durability of stents. It is a priceless tool for both patients and caregivers, providing actionable guidance on heart health monitoring as well as insights into the long-term prognosis and quality of life.

Overview of Angioplasty

A minimally invasive medical technique called an angioplasty is performed to treat clogged or narrowed blood vessels, usually arteries, in different body areas. Restoring blood flow via the damaged channel is the aim of angioplasty, which will enhance organ function and lessen symptoms like leg cramps and chest pain that are brought on by decreased blood flow.

Definition and Objective

A catheter with a balloon-like tip is used in angioplasty when it is placed into a blocked or narrowed blood artery. After the balloon is in place, it is inflated to widen the artery and restore blood flow by compressing the plaque accumulation against the arterial walls. After the balloon is deflated and removed, a stent—a tiny mesh tube—may also be implanted in certain instances to aid in maintaining the artery open.

Angioplasty's main goals are to relieve the symptoms of constricted or blocked arteries and lower the risk of problems like heart attacks and strokes that might result from decreased blood flow. Angioplasty can help patients live healthier, more active lifestyles and need fewer drugs to control their symptoms by increasing blood flow.

Evolution in History

The origins of angioplasty can be found in the middle of the 20th century when forward-thinking medical professionals started investigating methods for opening clogged arteries without requiring surgery. The first successful balloon angioplasty treatment was carried out in 1977 by Swiss cardiologist Dr. Andreas Gruentzig. Since then, advances in catheter and imaging technologies as well as the use of drug-eluting stents have improved the results of angioplasty procedures.

Angioplasty Types

There are various angioplasty techniques, each customized to the patient's unique requirements and the site of the clogged artery. Percutaneous coronary intervention (PCI), commonly referred to as coronary angioplasty, is a procedure performed to treat heart artery narrowing or blockage. Blocked arteries in the arms, legs, or other body regions outside the heart are the focus of peripheral angioplasty. By opening clogged arteries in the neck that feed blood to the brain, carotid angioplasty lowers the risk of stroke.

Other methods, such as atherectomy, which entails removing plaque from the artery using a specialized cutting tool, or laser angioplasty, which uses laser radiation to melt plaque, may be utilized during the treatment in addition to conventional balloon angioplasty.

Who Requires an Angioplasty?

If someone exhibits symptoms of decreased blood flow to the heart, brain, or extremities, such as shortness of breath, leg pain when walking, or chest pain, an angioplasty may be advised. It might also be recommended for people who have a history of smoking, high blood pressure, diabetes, or other conditions that put them at a higher risk of problems from constricted or clogged arteries.

Patients usually have diagnostic procedures, including angiography, before angioplasty to identify the position and extent of the blockage as well as to evaluate the general health of the blood arteries.

advantages for angioplasty

The less invasive nature of angioplasty, which lowers the dangers involved with open surgery and enables quicker recovery times, is one of its main advantages. A successful angioplasty can enhance overall quality of life by promptly relieving symptoms of decreased blood flow, such as leg cramps or chest pain.

Angioplasty can also lower the chance of major side effects, such as a heart attack, stroke, or limb amputation, by restoring blood flow through constricted or obstructed arteries, especially in people with underlying cardiovascular disease.

Furthermore, angioplasty may postpone or perhaps completely remove the need for more intrusive therapies like bypass surgery, as well as assist minimize the need for long-term medications to control symptoms, such as blood thinners or cholesterol-lowering medications.

CHAPTER ONE

THE CARDIAC VASCULAR SYSTEM'S ANATOMY AND PHYSIOLOGY

The circulatory system, also known as the cardiovascular system, is a sophisticated network that carries waste materials, nutrition, hormones, and oxygen throughout the body. The heart, a muscular organ the size of a fist that is situated somewhat to the left of the chest's center, is at the center of this system.

Heart's Structure

There are two atria and two ventricles, making up the four chambers of the heart. The pulmonary veins carry oxygenated blood from the lungs to the left atrium, while the superior and inferior vena cavae carry deoxygenated blood from the body to the right atrium. Following this, the atria constrict, forcing blood into the ventricles. While the left ventricle pumps blood that is rich in oxygen to the rest of the body, the right ventricle pumps blood that is deoxygenated to the lungs for oxygenation.

The Role Of Blood Vessels

The extensive network of blood vessels transports blood to and from the heart. Veins return blood that has lost oxygen from the body back to the heart, whereas arteries transport blood that is rich in oxygen from the heart to the body's tissues. The tiniest blood veins, called capillaries, help the blood and tissues exchange waste wastes and nutrition.

Coronary Arteries: An Overview

A vital component of the circulatory system, the coronary arteries provide the heart muscle with the nutrition and oxygen it needs to function. These arteries surround the heart and split off from the aorta to supply blood to every area of the heart muscle. Angina and heart attacks are among the heart disorders that can result from atherosclerosis, which narrows or blocks these arteries.

Circulation Of Blood Through The Heart

A specific route is followed by blood as it passes through the heart to guarantee effective circulation and oxygenation.

The superior and inferior vena cavae carry blood that has lost oxygen back to the body and return it to the heart through the right atrium. After that, it enters the right ventricle through the tricuspid valve and is pumped there by the pulmonary artery.

Blood absorbs oxygen and exhales carbon dioxide in the lungs, then travels back to the heart through the pulmonary veins and into the left atrium.

The left ventricle, which pumps oxygen-rich blood back into the body through the aorta, receives it after passing through the mitral valve.

Arterial Blockages' Effects

The accumulation of plaque in the arteries can lead to arterial blockages, which can have a major effect on cardiovascular health. Ischemic heart disease, which is typified by symptoms like angina pectoris or myocardial infarction (heart attack), can result from clogged arteries supplying the heart muscle. Similar to this, depending on the function of the affected organ, blockages in the arteries supplying other organs might cause a variety of health issues.

Recognizing the value of preserving heart health and avoiding ailments like artery blockages requires an understanding of the anatomy and physiology of the cardiovascular system. A healthy lifestyle that includes regular exercise, eating a balanced diet, and quitting smoking can help people lower their risk of cardiovascular disease and guarantee that their circulatory system is operating at its best.

CHAPTER TWO

CAUSES OF ARTERIAL BLOCKAGES AND THEIR SYMPTOMS

Atherosclerosis, another name for arterial blockages, is a condition in which fatty deposits accumulate inside the walls of arteries, narrowing the arteries and limiting blood flow. The buildup of fat, cholesterol, and other materials in the inner lining of the arteries is the main reason for arterial blockages. The accumulation of plaque causes the arteries to progressively harden and constrict, which lowers blood flow to the body's essential organs and tissues.

Arterial blockages are caused by several risk factors, including lifestyle decisions and heredity. Due to genetic factors, people who have a family history of heart disease or stroke are more likely to develop arterial blockages. Atherosclerosis can also be brought on by lifestyle decisions including smoking, drinking too much alcohol, eating poorly, and not exercising.

Depending on the blockage's location and degree, different artery blockages might cause different symptoms. Angina (chest pain or pressure), dyspnea, exhaustion, numbness, lightheadedness, and pain or discomfort in the arms, shoulders, neck, jaw, or back are typical symptoms. Severe arterial blockages may result in peripheral artery disease (PAD), which impairs limb blood flow, heart attack, or stroke.

Risk Variables (Hereditary, Lifestyle)

The likelihood of arterial blockages in an individual is mostly determined by genetic variables. You may have inherited genes that predispose you to atherosclerosis if there is a family history of heart disease or stroke. But your destiny is not solely determined by your genes. Lifestyle decisions are also very important in determining how artery blockages form and worsen.

Unhealthy lifestyle choices, such as eating a diet heavy in sodium, cholesterol, and saturated and trans fats, can exacerbate the accumulation of plaque in the arteries. Furthermore, being inactive can result in obesity, hypertension, and elevated cholesterol, all of which increase the risk of artery blockages. Another important risk factor that quickens the development of atherosclerosis is smoking, which damages the artery's inner lining and encourages the buildup of plaque.

Signs Of Obstructed Arteries

The location and degree of the obstruction can affect the symptoms of clogged arteries. Typical signs and symptoms include:

Angina, commonly known as chest pain or pressure, usually starts in the chest but can also spread to the arms, shoulders, neck, jaw, or back.

Breathing difficulties can be brought on by a decrease in blood supply to the heart or lungs.

Fatigue: Feeling drained or listless, particularly after exerting yourself, may indicate that the body is not getting enough blood to its tissues.

Weakness - A limited blood supply can result in muscle weakness, especially in the arms or legs.

Dizziness: Inadequate blood supply to the brain might cause lightheadedness or dizziness.

Pain or discomfort: People may feel pain or discomfort in their shoulders, back, neck, or jaw, particularly after exerting themselves physically or under stress.

How Obstacles Arise

Damage to the endothelium, the lining that lines the inside of the arteries, is the first step in the development of arterial blockages. Factors including smoking, diabetes, high blood pressure, excessive cholesterol, or inflammation can cause this harm. Substances including fat, cholesterol, calcium, and cellular waste products can build up in the artery walls once the endothelium is compromised.

These materials eventually combine to create plaque, which hardens and narrows the arteries to lessen blood flow. Plaque can eventually burst as it accumulates more material, forming blood clots that impede blood flow even more, or it might break off and migrate to other areas of the body, resulting in a heart attack or stroke. Arterial blockages frequently progress gradually and may not show symptoms until they are quite severe.

What Separates Stable From Unstable Plaques

A thick fibrous cap that surrounds the plaque and acts as stability and rupture prevention is a characteristic of stable plaques. When blood flow is partially blocked, these plaques can cause symptoms like intermittent claudication, or leg pain during walking. Typically, these plaques form slowly over time. Stable plaques, however, are less likely to result in unexpected consequences like a heart attack or stroke.

On the other hand, unstable plaques have a big lipid core that contains inflammatory cells and a thin fibrous cover that makes them more likely to rupture. Blood clots occur when an unstable plaque bursts, exposing the underlying tissue to blood and rapidly obstructing the artery, which can result in a heart attack or stroke. Unstable plaques frequently grow quickly and may not show any signs until a problem arises.

The Value Of Early Identification

To avoid consequences like peripheral artery disease, heart attacks, and strokes, early diagnosis of arterial blockages is essential. Regular health screenings can help identify risk factors and identify the presence of artery blockages before they create symptoms. These screenings can include blood pressure monitoring, cholesterol testing, and imaging studies like ultrasound or angiography.

Arterial blockages can be treated with lifestyle modifications like eating a heart-healthy diet, exercising frequently, giving up smoking, and taking care of underlying medical disorders like diabetes or high blood pressure. To lower the risk of problems in more severe cases, doctors may prescribe statins, antiplatelet medicines, or blood thinners.

In rare circumstances, operations like bypass surgery or angioplasty might be required to restore blood flow to the damaged arteries. While bypass surgery includes making a new conduit for blood to avoid the clogged artery, angioplasty is pumping a balloon-like device inside the artery to enlarge it and enhance blood flow. For those with artery blockages, early detection and intervention can greatly enhance outcomes and quality of life.

CHAPTER THREE

DIAGNOSTIC METHODOLOGIES

Non-Invasive Examinations (Stress Test, EKG)

The diagnostic process for cardiac diseases, particularly those requiring angioplasty, heavily relies on non-invasive testing. The Electrocardiogram, sometimes known as the EKG or ECG, is a prominent instrument among these diagnostics. Electrodes are affixed to your arms, legs, and chest to record the electrical activity of your heart. The procedure is painless. This aids in identifying irregular cardiac rhythms and heart attack warning signals.

Stress testing is a more popular non-invasive test. You will be required to exercise under observation on a stationary bike or treadmill for this test. This gives medical professionals important information about possible coronary artery blockages and how your heart functions under stress. It's similar to exercising your heart in a safe setting to observe how it reacts.

Imaging Methods (MRI, CT Angiography)

Imaging methods are essential for the diagnosis of cardiac diseases, particularly for determining the degree of coronary artery blockages. The use of CT angiography is one such method.

It entails giving yourself a bloodstream injection of contrast dye and getting precise X-ray images of your heart. This aids in the identification of artery blockages and narrowing, directing subsequent treatment choices.

Another effective method for diagnosing heart problems is magnetic resonance imaging or MRI. Without utilizing radiation, it offers finely detailed images of the heart and blood vessels. An MRI can identify structural and functional problems in the heart, which can assist medical professionals in determining whether an angioplasty is necessary. It's especially helpful in determining how well the heart pumps blood and identifying any cardiac muscle injury.

Invasive Exams (Coronary Angiography)

Invasive examinations like coronary angiography are required to diagnose cardiac diseases when non-invasive testing is insufficient. To perform this surgery, a catheter must be threaded through a blood vessel, typically in the wrist or groin, and a contrast dye must be injected straight into the coronary arteries. After that, X-ray pictures are obtained to see any obstructions or constricted regions.

With the use of coronary angiography, cardiologists can assess your coronary arteries in real-time and choose the best course of action, including angioplasty.

Coronary angiography is regarded as the gold standard for diagnosing coronary artery disease and directing interventional therapies, despite being more intrusive than non-invasive testing.

Biomarkers And Blood Tests

When it comes to identifying cardiac disorders and determining the likelihood of consequences like heart attacks, blood testing is essential.

Damage to heart muscle cells releases biomarkers into the bloodstream, such as troponin and creatine kinase-MB (CK-MB). Increased concentrations of these biomarkers point to potential cardiac damage, which could result from unstable angina or a heart attack.

Blood tests examine cholesterol levels in addition to biomarkers, which is crucial information for determining your risk of coronary artery disease. Elevated low-density lipoprotein (LDL) cholesterol, commonly known as "bad" cholesterol, can cause plaque to accumulate in the arteries, raising the risk of heart attacks and strokes. Keeping an eye on cholesterol levels aids in the treatment and prevention of heart disease.

Interpreting The Findings Of A Diagnosis

A thorough comprehension of the various tests and their implications is necessary for interpreting the findings of diagnostic procedures. To create a comprehensive picture of the patient's cardiovascular health, data from non-invasive testing, imaging investigations, invasive treatments, and blood tests must be analyzed.

To guarantee an accurate diagnosis and efficient treatment planning, cardiologists, radiologists, and other healthcare specialists must work together during this procedure.

Healthcare professionals take into account various criteria when interpreting diagnostic data, including the degree of heart muscle damage, the presence and severity of coronary artery blockages, and the overall risk of consequences. In addition, they consider the patient's symptoms, medical history, and heart disease risk factors.

Using a comprehensive approach, treatment plans can be customized to fit the specific requirements of each patient, taking into account changes to lifestyle, prescription drugs, or invasive procedures like angioplasty.

CHAPTER FOUR

EXPLAINED: THE ANGIOPLASTY PROCEDURE

Angioplasty is a minimally invasive treatment used to open restricted or blocked arteries. It is often referred to as balloon angioplasty or percutaneous transluminal angioplasty (PTA).

It is frequently carried out to increase blood flow to various body areas impacted by peripheral artery disease (PAD) or to restore blood flow to the heart in situations of coronary artery disease (CAD). This surgery helps relieve symptoms such as angina (chest discomfort), dyspnea, and pain in the legs from decreased blood flow.

Methodical Procedure

Preparation: You will receive instructions regarding medicine and fasting before the surgery. Once you and your healthcare team have discussed the advantages and disadvantages, you will need to sign a consent form. Throughout the surgery, an intravenous (IV) line will be placed into your arm to deliver fluids and drugs.

Anesthesia: To make the place where the catheter will be implanted, usually in the groin or wrist, numb, you will be given a local anesthetic. To aid with relaxation, you could occasionally additionally receive a small amount of medication.

Catheter insertion: A tiny skin incision is made, and a flexible, thin tube known as a catheter is placed into an artery. The catheter is carefully threaded through the arteries until it reaches the blockage site, guided by X-ray imaging.

Angiography: A particular dye is administered through the catheter as soon as it reaches the artery that is damaged. With the use of this dye, the interventional cardiologist can precisely determine the location and degree of obstruction on X-ray pictures.

Balloon inflation involves inserting a small, deflated balloon that is connected to a catheter into the constricted artery once the blockage has been identified.

After that, the balloon is inflated, which widens the opening for blood flow and presses the plaque up against the arterial walls.

Placement of Stent (if necessary): To assist keep the newly expanded artery open, a tiny metal mesh tube known as a stent may occasionally be implanted.

By offering support and preventing the artery from collapsing or being blocked again, the stent functions as a scaffold.

Completion Angiography: Following the procedure, a further angiography round may be conducted to verify that blood flow has improved and that no problems, such as dissections or residual obstructions, have occurred.

Closure: To stop the bleeding, the catheter is finally taken out and pressure is applied to the incision site. To promote healing, the area may be covered with a bandage or compression device.

Tools And Apparatus Employed

The following are the main instruments and apparatus used in angioplasty:

Catheters: Flexible, thin tubes that are used to enter and exit the arteries.

Guidewires: Tiny wires that are passed through the catheter to aid in vascular voyaging.

Balloons: To expand constricted arteries, tiny inflatable balloons are affixed to the catheter.

Stents: Reinforced metal mesh tubes that keep newly enlarged arteries from constricting.

X-ray machines and contrast dye are utilized as part of the angiography equipment, which helps to see the arteries.

The interventional cardiologist's role

An important function of the interventional cardiologist is to carry out angioplasty operations. These highly skilled professionals are proficient in the diagnosis and treatment of cardiovascular diseases with the least amount of intrusive procedures.

The interventional cardiologist oversees every step of the angioplasty process, including balloon inflation, angiography, and catheter insertion.

To maximize results, they also have to make important judgments on the use of stents and any other procedures that could be required.

What Takes Place Throughout The Process

You will be sedated but conscious during the angioplasty procedure, and you might experience some pressure or slight discomfort as the catheter is inserted and advanced through your arteries. Throughout the surgery, you will be attentively observed for any indications of potential complications, such as bleeding or abnormal cardiac rhythms. After angioplasty, the majority of patients report significant symptom improvement; however, individual results may differ based on the degree of artery blockage and general health.

Following a procedure

Following angioplasty, you'll be taken to a recovery area so that your health indicators can be watched. To promote healing at the insertion site and lessen the chance of bleeding, you will need to remain motionless for a few hours.

Your medical team will provide you with information on how to take care of your incision site, including how to keep it dry and clean. Medication may be administered to you to lower your risk of problems and avoid blood clots.

You will be arranged for follow-up appointments so that we can keep an eye on your progress and evaluate how well the operation worked to improve blood flow and relieve your symptoms.

It is crucial to adhere to your physician's advice on lifestyle modifications, such as giving up smoking, maintaining a heart-healthy diet, and getting regular exercise, to preserve the advantages of angioplasty and lower your chance of experiencing another cardiovascular event.

CHAPTER FIVE

DANGERS AND COMMITMENTS

Like any medical operation, angioplasty has certain dangers and problems that should be considered. Knowing these risks can help you plan and make an educated decision about what to expect before, during, and after the treatment.

Typical Risks

Among the most frequent hazards of angioplasty are bleeding and infection. There is a chance of bleeding during the surgery since a little incision is made to access the blood vessels. Even while this is typically not serious and may be handled by the medical staff, there are situations when it might need further care or observation.

Another possible risk is infection, however this is not very common. The medical team sterilizes equipment and uses antibiotics when needed to reduce the danger of infection. After the treatment, it's crucial to watch out for any indications of infection, such as increasing redness, swelling, or pain at the incision site.

Uncommon Problems

Although angioplasty operations are generally safe, a small number of uncommon problems may arise. These include heart attacks and strokes, however they are not common. A blood clot that forms during the procedure may travel to the brain and obstruct blood vessels, increasing the risk of stroke. In a similar vein, a blood clot blocking a coronary artery can cause a heart attack by preventing blood flow to the heart muscle.

Even though these issues are uncommon, it's important to recognize the warning signs and symptoms. To reduce the chance of these issues, the medical team will continuously monitor you both during and after the treatment. If a problem does arise, they will move quickly to address it.

How Hazards Are Handled

Before, during, and after the treatment, the medical team takes several steps to manage the risks related to angioplasty. You will get a comprehensive evaluation before the surgery to determine any factors that may raise your risk of complications and to examine your general health. This could involve a review of your medical history, radiological scans, and blood testing.

The medical staff will keep a careful eye on your vital signs throughout the surgery and take appropriate action if something goes wrong. They might give you medicine to control your blood pressure and heart rate, or they might prevent blood clots. You will be closely observed in the recovery area following the procedure to make sure you are stable and that no issues arise.

Signs of Difficulties to Be Aware of

It's critical to recognize the warning signs and symptoms of potential complications following angioplasty. Among them are:

elevated discomfort, edema, or redness where the incision is made

Breathing Problems Or Chest Pain

One-sided weakness or numbness in the body

alterations in speech or vision

lightheadedness or fainting

It's critical to get medical attention right away if you encounter any of these symptoms. The optimum result can be ensured and issues can be kept from getting worse with prompt treatment.

When To Get Medical Assistance

It's critical to your recovery from angioplasty to know when to seek medical attention. Do not hesitate to call your doctor or visit the closest emergency department if you encounter any of the following symptoms:

continuous pressure or pain in the chest

Breathing difficulties or shortness of breath

severe vertigo or headache

Loss of awareness or fainting

Redness, swelling, or discharge where the incision was made

These signs may point to a problem that needs to be treated right away. Don't brush them off or think they will go away by themselves. Getting therapy as soon as possible will help avoid major issues and guarantee a full recovery following angioplasty.

CHAPTER SIX

REPAY AND RESUMMATION

It makes sense to be curious about the healing process following an angioplasty procedure. Thankfully, recovery for most people is rather uneventful.

To guarantee the best possible healing and avoid complications, it's imperative that you carefully adhere to your doctor's recommendations.

Usually, the first stage of recovery happens in the hospital, where doctors will attentively check your condition. It's natural to feel a little sore or uncomfortable where the incision was made. Painkillers might assist in reducing any discomfort you may have.

Your healthcare staff will offer direction on progressively increasing your level of exercise as you move through the rehabilitation process. Even though it's critical to take it easy and let your body repair itself at first, an extended period of inactivity can hinder your recuperation.

Walking is one of the lightest exercises that can assist increase blood circulation and aid in the healing process.

Throughout the healing phase, your healthcare practitioner will also provide you with advice on how to manage your medications and food.

To maintain your cardiovascular health and avert further issues, it is imperative that you carefully adhere to these recommendations.

It's critical to address the psychological and emotional parts of healing in addition to the physical. An angioplasty may be a major event that causes a range of feelings, such as worry or anxiety. During this period, getting emotional support from loved ones or joining a support group might be helpful.

Quick Post-Procedure Treatment

You will be attentively observed in a hospital recovery unit immediately after angioplasty. This monitoring guarantees that any possible issues can be resolved quickly. Your vital signs will be monitored and your overall health will be evaluated by healthcare professionals while you are in the recovery area.

Due to the anesthesia or sedative used during the treatment, you might feel a little groggy or sleepy. This is typical and will go away in a few hours. You could occasionally need to spend the night in the hospital to be observed, particularly if there were any issues with the procedure.

You must adhere to your healthcare provider's guidelines for activity and movement during this period. It could be suggested that you stay away from certain motions or activities that might put tension on the incision site. Your healthcare staff will also provide you with information on wound care and pain control.

It's critical that you quickly let your healthcare provider know about any worries or symptoms you notice. This can include breathing difficulties, bleeding profusely, chest pain, or infection at the location of the incision. A smooth recovery can be encouraged and complications can be avoided with early detection and action.

Hospital Discharge Procedure

After angioplasty, the hospital discharge procedure signifies the change from inpatient to outpatient care. Your medical team will make sure you are stable and ready to continue recovering at home before releasing you.

During the discharge procedure, you will be given instructions on wound care, medication management, and activity limits. Before you leave the hospital, it is important to get any questions you may have answered and any doubts cleared up. Your medical staff is available to support you and answer any questions you may have regarding your recuperation.

You will also be given information regarding follow-up visits and post-discharge care before you leave the hospital. These consultations are crucial for tracking your development and resolving any problems that could come up while you're recovering.

It is crucial that you carefully adhere to the discharge instructions that your healthcare team has given you once you are at home.

This includes taking prescription drugs as directed, abstaining from physically demanding activities, and keeping an eye out for any changes or worsening of your symptoms.

Medication And Appointments For Follow-Up

Your doctor may recommend medicine after an angioplasty to assist you manage your condition and lower the chance of problems. Blood thinners, cholesterol-lowering pharmaceuticals, and blood pressure meds are a few examples of these medications.

You must take these drugs precisely as directed by your doctor. Medication errors or sudden stops can impede your healing and raise your risk of problems.

You will be given medication and made appointments for follow-up visits with your healthcare practitioner. These consultations are crucial for tracking your development, evaluating the efficacy of your care, and resolving any possible problems or concerns.

Your healthcare practitioner may assess your cardiovascular health during these visits by ordering procedures like imaging studies or blood testing.

To guarantee the best possible results, your treatment plan may need to be modified in light of the findings of these tests.

Guidelines For Physical Activity

After angioplasty, physical activity is essential to the healing process. Even while it's crucial to take it easy and give your body time to recuperate, you can enhance your general health and cardiovascular health by gradually increasing your activity level.

Personalized recommendations for physical exercise will be given by your healthcare professional based on your unique situation and general health. Generally speaking, it is advised to begin with mild exercises like walking and progressively increase the duration and intensity.

When exercising, it's critical to pay attention to your body and refrain from exerting yourself too much. Stop exercising right away and get medical help if you have any of the following symptoms: dizziness, shortness of breath, chest pain, or other worrisome symptoms.

Strength training and flexibility exercises, in addition to aerobic activity, can assist enhance cardiovascular health and general fitness. To be sure it's safe and suitable for your condition, it's crucial to speak with your healthcare physician before beginning any new fitness regimen.

Mental And Emotional Assistance

An important life event like having an angioplasty can cause a range of feelings, such as dread, uncertainty, or anxiety. It is imperative to attend to the emotional and psychological dimensions of healing to promote general health and recuperation.

Seeking out emotional support from friends, family, or a support group can help reduce anxiety or feelings of loneliness. Talking to people who have had similar operations done about your experiences can provide important perspective and support.

In addition, if you find it difficult to manage the psychological or emotional effects of angioplasty, you might want to speak with a mental health expert. Therapy or counseling can offer a secure setting for you to explore your emotions, pick up coping mechanisms, and strengthen your ability to bounce back from setbacks.

Recall that emotional and psychological as well as bodily healing occurs. Taking good care of your mental and emotional health is crucial to your recuperation and can assist you in overcoming the obstacles that come with living after angioplasty.

CHAPTER SEVEN

CHANGES IN LIFESTYLE AFTER ANGIOPLASTY

The Value Of A Balanced Diet

Following an angioplasty, eating a balanced diet is crucial to preserving cardiovascular health. The main components of a heart-healthy diet include usually whole grains, fruits, vegetables, lean meats, and healthy fats. These foods are full of nutrients that assist in maintaining heart health generally and control blood pressure, weight, and cholesterol.

Making a point of including a range of vibrant fruits and vegetables in meals guarantees that the body is getting enough vitamins, minerals, and antioxidants. These nutrients are essential for lowering inflammation, enhancing blood vessel health, and fending against oxidative stress, all of which can hasten the course of heart disease.

Fiber from whole grains, such as quinoa, brown rice, and oats, helps decrease cholesterol and increase satiety, both of which support weight management. Lean protein options like fish, chicken, beans, and legumes can assist in lowering the consumption of saturated fat, which is further beneficial to heart health, as opposed to red meat.

For the heart to continue functioning at its best, a diet rich in foods like avocados, almonds, seeds, and olive oil must contain healthy fats. These fats, in particular monounsaturated and polyunsaturated fats, can reduce the risk of plaque accumulation in the arteries by raising HDL (good) cholesterol levels and lowering LDL (bad) cholesterol levels.

After angioplasty, it's also a good idea to limit your intake of processed foods, sugary snacks, and beverages with added sugar. These products have the potential to cause inflammation, weight gain, and insulin resistance—all conditions that are harmful to heart health. Choosing home-cooked meals that are produced with whole, fresh foods instead of premade ones gives you more control over how much nutrition you consume and improves your general health.

Following angioplasty, implementing these dietary modifications into daily life can greatly enhance cardiovascular health outcomes and lower the chance of subsequent cardiac events. By emphasizing nutrient-dense foods and reducing consumption of processed and unhealthy options, people can improve their quality of life and aid in their recovery.

Follow Exercise Guidelines

Those who have had angioplasty should be physically active regularly to support their general health and cardiovascular health. Exercise benefits cardiac muscle strength, circulation, blood pressure regulation, weight management, and mood enhancement.

Reintroducing exercise to one's regimen after angioplasty should be done gradually and under the supervision of medical professionals. Low-impact exercises like swimming, cycling, or walking can help restore strength and endurance while lowering the chance of strain or injury.

People can gradually raise the duration and intensity of their workouts as their fitness levels rise. Including strength training, flexibility training, and aerobic workouts in a weekly regimen can improve overall physical health and offer comprehensive cardiovascular advantages.

Aim for at least 150 minutes per week, spaced out over many days, of moderate-intensity aerobic activity or 75 minutes of vigorous-intensity aerobic activity. Furthermore, including strength training activities that focus on large muscle groups two or three times a week might enhance general functional capacity, metabolism, and muscular tone.

Pay attention to your body and modify the level of activity as necessary, especially if you're feeling tired or uncomfortable. Finding the right balance between pushing oneself to increase one's level of fitness and avoiding strain or overexertion is crucial because these actions could jeopardize recuperation and general health.

When it comes to continuing an exercise regimen after angioplasty, consistency is essential. Maintaining motivation and sticking to a regular workout schedule is much easier when interesting and sustainable activities are found. Finding activities that suit personal interests and preferences encourages long-term adherence to an active lifestyle, whether that means playing leisure sports, going on brisk walks outdoors, or enrolling in group fitness courses.

Through the implementation of a diverse range of exercises and a regular physical activity regimen, individuals can achieve optimal cardiovascular health, elevate their overall fitness levels, and experience an improved quality of life following angioplasty.

Quitting Smoking

One of the most important lifestyle adjustments people may make after angioplasty to enhance cardiovascular health and lower the chance of problems in the future is probably quitting smoking. Smoking cigarettes is linked to a higher risk of heart attacks, strokes, and other cardiovascular events. It is also a key risk factor for coronary artery disease.

Giving up smoking dramatically increases lung function, improves circulation, and lowers the risk of future damage to the heart and blood vessels. People may see improvements in their breathing, circulation, and energy levels within a few weeks of quitting, which paves the way for improved long-term health outcomes.

After angioplasty, there are several tools and techniques to assist with quitting smoking. Successful quitting can be facilitated by the use of nicotine replacement therapies, including patches, gum, lozenges, and prescription drugs, which can help control cravings and withdrawal symptoms.

Throughout the stopping process, behavioral counseling, support groups, and smoking cessation programs provide invaluable direction, accountability, and encouragement. These materials give people the methods, techniques, and networks of support they need to beat their addiction to nicotine and stay smoke-free for the long term.

Successful smoking cessation requires recognizing and resolving the stressors and triggers that lead to smoking behavior. People can better manage cravings and temptations by learning coping methods, identifying non-tobacco smoke stress-relieving techniques, and creating a supportive atmosphere.

After angioplasty, patients must stick with their smoking cessation plans and get additional support as needed. While relapse is normal during the quitting process, it's important to remember that setbacks are transient and should not be interpreted as failures. People who are determined, persistent, and supported can overcome their addiction to nicotine and reap the many health advantages of leading a smoke-free lifestyle.

Individuals can greatly lower their risk of cardiovascular problems, improve overall health outcomes, and improve their quality of life by making quitting smoking a priority after angioplasty.

Stress Reduction

After angioplasty, effective stress management is essential to lowering the risk of subsequent cardiac episodes and enhancing general well-being. Long-term stress can exacerbate cardiovascular health problems such as high blood pressure, inflammation, improper coping mechanisms, and others.

People can develop a sense of calm, resilience, and emotional well-being as well as improve their ability to handle stress by implementing stress-reduction strategies and lifestyle habits. Examples of relaxation techniques that can help induce relaxation and lower stress levels include progressive muscle relaxation, guided imagery, mindfulness meditation, and deep breathing exercises.

Frequent exercise, such as tai chi, yoga, or walking, can also be an effective way to decrease stress because it improves mood, releases endorphins, and encourages relaxation. Additional channels for stress release and emotional expression can be found in artistic endeavors, hobbies, and fulfilling social interactions.

Putting self-care first and establishing limits to avoid burnout is critical to post-angioplasty stress management. This can entail planning regular downtime, assigning responsibilities to others, declining overly demanding obligations, and, if necessary, asking friends, family, or medical experts for assistance.

Healthy coping mechanisms like problem-solving, positive reframing, and reaching out to others for support can make it easier for people to get through difficult times and develop resilience in the face of hardship.

It's critical to identify rising stress levels and act quickly to alleviate them before they have a detrimental effect on one's health and well-being.

People can lessen the negative effects of stress on their cardiovascular health, boost their overall quality of life, speed up their recovery, and improve their long-term prognosis by adopting stress-reduction tactics, lifestyle changes, and good coping mechanisms in their everyday lives after angioplasty.

Routine Check-Ups With The Doctor

Following angioplasty, patients must undergo routine medical examinations to monitor their cardiovascular health, evaluate the effectiveness of their therapy, and identify any potential risks or consequences as soon as possible. These examinations offer healthcare professionals important chances to assess the efficacy of therapeutic initiatives and modify the care plan as needed.

Healthcare professionals may conduct a variety of tests and evaluations to examine cardiovascular health markers such as blood pressure, cholesterol, and heart function during medical check-ups. Electrocardiograms (ECGs), echocardiograms, stress tests, blood tests, and imaging examinations like CT scans or angiography are a few examples of these.

Medical check-ups give healthcare professionals the chance to address lifestyle issues, medication adherence, and any worries or inquiries patients may have regarding their recovery and ongoing care, in addition to evaluating physical health.

The optimization of health outcomes and resolution of any potential obstacles or problems necessitate candid communication and cooperation between patients and healthcare providers.

Medical check-ups may be planned at regular intervals, such as every three to six months initially, then annually, or biannually thereafter, depending on individual needs and risk factors.

However, depending on a patient's unique situation, the results of their therapy, and the advice of their healthcare professional, the number and timing of checkups may change.

Following an angioplasty, patients must prioritize going to their planned doctor's appointments and following any advice given by their medical team. Regular check-ups are essential for maintaining cardiovascular health and general well-being because they enable continuous monitoring, preventive care, and prompt intervention when necessary.

Proactively scheduling follow-up appointments and keeping lines of communication open with medical professionals can help patients better manage their cardiovascular health after angioplasty, reduce the chance of problems, and live longer.

CHAPTER EIGHT

QUESTIONS ASKED REGULARLY

What Is The Stent's Duration Of Use?

A stent's duration can vary based on several factors, such as the kind of stent that is utilized, the patient's general health, and lifestyle choices. Drug-eluting stents (DES) often have a longer lifespan than bare-metal stents (BMS). By releasing medication to stop blockages from recurring, DES may be able to extend the stent's life. DES can, in most cases, endure for many years, or even a lifetime, provided the patient leads a healthy lifestyle and complies with their doctor's advice.

It's crucial to realize, though, that a stent is not a permanent solution. Restenosis, or the re-narrowing of the artery as a result of the accumulation of plaque or scar tissue, is a possibility over time. Scheduling routine follow-up consultations with your cardiologist is essential for keeping an eye on the stent's condition and quickly addressing any issues.

Can Blockages Happen Again?

Indeed, obstructions may return even following angioplasty and stent implantation. This possibility emphasizes how crucial it is to live a heart-healthy lifestyle and use prescription drugs as directed. Recurrence of blockages can be caused by several factors, including diabetes, high blood pressure, excessive cholesterol, and smoking. As such, it's critical to successfully manage these risk factors through adherence to medication, lifestyle changes, and routine check-ups with your healthcare professional.

If blockages recur or grow new ones, patients may occasionally need further treatments like coronary artery bypass surgery or repeat angioplasty. That being said, there are hazards associated with these treatments as well, so it's important to talk about the best course of action with your healthcare team.

influence on day-to-day activities and lives

By reducing symptoms like chest pain or shortness of breath, angioplasty and stent placement can greatly enhance the quality of life for a large number of patients. It is common to encounter certain restrictions or modifications after the operation, nevertheless.

To allow the artery to heal properly, your healthcare professional may advise rest and limited physical activity following angioplasty. To lower the risk of problems and avoid blood clots, you might also need to take medicine.

Following your doctor's instructions, progressively resume your daily routine of physical exercise while you heal. After the treatment, you can usually return to your regular activities, such as working out and going to work, a few days to a few weeks later. But it's important to pay attention to your body and not overextend yourself, particularly when you're first recovering.

How To Keep An Eye On Your Heart Health

After angioplasty, keeping an eye on your heart health is essential to avoiding problems and preserving general health. Regular follow-up appointments are likely to be advised by your healthcare practitioner to evaluate your progress, keep an eye on the stent's status, and modify your treatment plan as necessary.

Apart from routine medical examinations, there are other actions you may take daily to keep an eye on the health of your heart. If you have diabetes, keep an eye on your blood pressure, cholesterol, and blood sugar levels as they can have an impact on the condition of your arteries. To keep your heart healthy and your arteries clear, eat a balanced diet low in saturated fats, cholesterol, and sodium and get frequent exercise.

Be mindful of any health changes or symptoms, such as exhaustion, shortness of breath, or chest pain, and notify your healthcare practitioner right away. You may lower your risk of problems and improve your quality of life by being proactive and watchful about your heart health.

Prognosis Over The Long Term And Quality Of Life

After angioplasty and stent implantation, the long-term prognosis is usually good, particularly when lifestyle changes and continued medical care are included. Numerous patients report notable improvements in their quality of life and symptoms, which enables them to lead busy and satisfying lives.

But it's crucial to understand that cardiovascular disease is a chronic illness that needs to be managed for the rest of one's life. This entails adhering to prescription guidelines, scheduling frequent follow-up visits, and adopting a healthy lifestyle to stop blockages and difficulties from recurring.

A high standard of living can be sustained for many years by people who receive the right care and follow their doctors' advice. But to maximize your long-term prognosis and general well-being, you must remain knowledgeable, proactive, and involved in your healthcare.

www.ingramcontent.com/pod-product-compliance
Lightning Source LLC
Chambersburg PA
CBHW071841210526
45479CB00001B/231